FOOD SICK NATION
OUR OBSESSIVE RELATIONSHIP WITH FOOD

Authors note:
In the following, I talk about hating myself. Wanting to hurt myself and why I believe we need to reevaluate our relationship with food.
With that said, the feelings that I speak of are not ease to overcome and not to be taken lightly. And the very real impact of obsession and addiction requires more attention then a book can provide.

Which is to say, this book and its concepts are not mental health or medical advice. And if you are one of the millions of people struggling with the notion of hurting themselves in any way, please put this down and get help.

You do not have to be alone.
Please contact the number below.

National Suicide Prevention Lifeline
800-273-8255

ob·ses·sion

An idea or thought that continually
preoccupies or intrudes on a person's
mind.

FOOD SICK NATION

ONE
THE APPETIZER

There is nothing more destructive to our health or our planet than our sick relationship with food.
Not empty calories.
Not GMO or hybrid foods.
Not chemical injected food.
Not coal tar coloring or known carcinogens, additives or preservatives....
Nothing.
Not that you should eat any of that but still if you did....it would not be as big an issue.
The truth is that if we had anything close to a healthy understanding of how we should be thinking about food, we would never eat that shit anyway.

Like someone saying that you need a lot of OJ when your coming off heroine. When if you never took a hot batch in your arm... the need for the OJ would be moot.

And in many ways, that's just what we do.
Create crisis, sickness and obsession and
then use other poison as a cure.
**Like an insane, self inflicted form of
munchausen by proxy.**

**Eat, drink, gain, exercise, starve,
punish, lose, repeat.**

From outside looking in...it might seem to
a newcomer to our world that we are
completely fucking mad.

No one knows more about this cycle and
how we abuse ourselves over food then
me.
I have been dragging around a dead fat
man for over 35 years. A 130 pound dead
weight clingy slob.
Unwanted and unloved is he yet he would
not go away.
I have fought him.
Fed him.
Wished him dead and gone.
Cried over him, tried to pack him into
pants 2 sizes too small and loathed the
both of us for the first 35 years of my life.

And while that is a sick and sad story.... it
is literally a common one.
Which is the most intolerable cruelty of all.

I have committed to losing him over and over. Like a drunk. Making a deal with god in the bathroom on the morning after. Begging for help. For the pain to go away. Making promises that no sane person would ever believe.

I have gone shopping.
Hauled a pile of pants and shirts into the dressing room. Only to be overcome with flop sweat, anger and a form of silent debilitating embarrassment as nothing fit.

Alone in a 5 by 5 box, crying like a baby. Feeling that if I did not have so many people depending on me, that I might just give up.
Having to do the walk of shame as I replace the shit that I can't buy on the racks.
Knowing full well that everyone was looking at me. Laughing at the fat guy that could not find a tent big enough for his ass.
Creating a narrative in my head should anyone ask if I was alright.
A few basic excuses like "I forgot my wallet" or "I'm late for work".

You know, the kind of sick shit that crazy people must do when they know they are not normal but are trying to fit in.

Then, waddling out of the store, hearing the sound of my own thighs rubbing together as I walk. Begging for the sound to stop. To go away, less someone hear it too. You see, I know it's happening. That's why I was there to begin with.
Because all of my pants have holes in there.
In the inter thighs. The lasting scares of the fat and its assault on the few pairs of pants I forced myself to find.
The unseen and imaginary eyes on me burn as I head for safety of the car.
And then?
Finding myself in the parking lot of Burger king, attempting a form of culinary suicide.
Hows that for a real and honest confession? And to be clear, I am still in recovery. I have to work on it everyday. Just like any addict.
To stop myself from falling back into the cycles that sought to destroy my younger life. I would spare you that if I could.
And I suppose I should have put this next thing on the book cover but: THIS IS NOT A WEIGHT LOSS BOOK.

Think of it as the first contact with a person that is outside the cult you were born into. Contact with a person just like you. Yet, I am not the same anymore.

And again, full disclosure – I am not thin!
I am what you could be.

Now, just who the hell am I?
Well, by the account above, I am a person
that hated themselves. That had a sick
and obsessive dependency on the thing
that they hated.
But just how did I get here?
I beat this demon with knowledge.
By learning shit and knowing shit.

Seeing the truth in the world around us.
And listening to the non-stop
conversations about food that is literally
everywhere, 24-7-365.
Pounded at us.
Driven into us and is, pardon the pun,
force fed to us by everyone.

And by listing to those people around me
when they said they loved me. I found my
love for my self there. In those that
depended on me and trusted me.
Later, I came to understand that it was
not about how I looked on the outside that
mattered. It was what I put inside me that
really mattered.
A thing that everyone knows in the
abstract but, simply can not come to hold
as "truth one".

And I could be healthy and happy, even if
I never killed and buried that fat guy I was
hauling around the world.

Why did I tell you this?
Simple.
I wanted you to know that I am not
someone that is just selling you
something.
A person that read some book and lost 10
pounds once and now thinks that their
personal story can be monetized and is
one of importance and motivation.

My only motivation is to help you.
Perhaps free you.
And to make a point that no one has
seemed to make -

The way we eat is not just killing us it's killing the planet!

And so that you will know that I know,
first hand, what I am talking about when
I say we have a relationship problem with
food. This sick and obsessive relationship
with food.

And that sucks because food is important.

TWO
The Primer

Where necessity ends and abuse begins

How important is food?

That is a loaded question for sure. We all know that without food we die. And on the way there, we suffer.
However, where is the line between need and abuse? And how do we sort out all of the things we have been told from what is real and true and healthy?

Past that, the impact from the world around us and the impact from our whole lives with food. From the feeling of home that food brings.

The feelings that we associate with eating with family and friends and the all encompassing experience of that perfect holiday meal.

And beyond that, food itself, has strong effects on our brains. The chemical reactions we have from ingesting food is hard to identify and even harder to give up. Ask anyone, they would gladly give up smoking over pizza!
And as a past smoker, I got that wonderful experience to drawn on too.
Both of them.

Then there is the social aspect of food. Meeting people. Filling time. Taking a break from the work day. Rewarding ourselves for a job well done or a hard day.

No doubt about it – we are less food consumers then we are food users.

And the truth is that while you can be sure that someone will, without solicitation, give you the good advice to quit smoking. There is no widespread disdain for food.

You would be far more likely to have a total stranger come up to you and ask you where you got that yummy looking doughnut! And then tell you about their favorite pastry shop.

Like two junkies talking about where to buy the best drugs!

And the only reason we do not look at it that way is...because when everybody is getting high – no one has a drug problem!

The abuse of food is normal now. Legal and encouraged!

Which is to say, the point where need ends and abuse begins happened long before you and I were born. That ship sailed shortly after Columbus!

The point where hunger was replaced by cravings is a distant fuzzy image.
We are far past that now.

And while one could argue that having an abundance of food help us become who we are.
It fed us and helped us along the way to ruling the world. In many ways it has become our cross to bare.
And lastly, half of the world still goes to bed hungry each night - while we throw away millions of tons of good food every day.
And, yes, wasting food is a form of abuse.

All offered as evidence that we have a historically strange relationship with food. We have gone from staving and needing to gluttony and waste in under 5000 years.

Yet we have never been Ok with what we have.
Never has the primal urge to eat, store, seek and fed in case of famine subsided.

Instead, we have changed the reasons for the importance of food. Once important to survive now has become what one could only call a "food lifestyle".

**Or as the old cliche goes;
"Living to eat rather then eating to live"**

so, now, how is food important?

Well by all accounts it is second only to money in our cultures. And as you will see – food is money. A whole shit load of it!

It's so important we have 2 rooms in our homes totally dedicated to it and a few storage areas.

.

The most expensive equipment we own surrounds food. From the refrigerator to stove, microwave, there are over 65 appliances to cook food with. And hundreds of preparation devices. As is eating, cleaning, and storage of utensils.

In fact, more time and consideration in design goes into a kitchen and dinning room then any other part of the home.

Bathrooms are just slapped together and bedrooms follow one simply rule – make them big enough for the bed.
But the kitchen?
Time and thought.
And why not.
Its the big deal in the house.

Some people are lucky enough to have an eat in kitchen, that way you are never even a few feet from more food.

We have pantries and closets filled with dry goods and even freezers filled to the top in the garage. And depending on the size of the home, a second "wet bar" with a smaller refrigerator in the basement or another in garage is needed too.
As if all the store will close tomorrow when the war starts!

Like there will be some massive cow
rapture or chicken apocalypse at any
moment.

We live in a world of supersonic jets,
space travel and unprecedented
transportation of goods yet we are hording
for the end times.
Its troubling when you look at this way.
And this is the only way to look at it. You
can try to pass it off as a personal
freedom issue but...your just kidding
yourself.
And here's why.

As of 2020, there were over 1million
restaurants in the country.
Over 63,000 grocery stores.
And at least 36,000 manufacturers for
food products.
And a colossal 148,000 convenience stores
for snacks and bad food. And those
numbers grow every year.

There is a road in Florida that runs from
Stuart Florida to Miami and there is a
50,000 square foot Publix or Winn Dixie
grocery store on that street every few
miles!
For a hundred miles!!!!

And lets not forget that you do not need to go to any of these places to get something in your mouth.
You can get hordes of bubble sugar water and corn syrup filled candy at hardware stores, gas station, office buildings, street vendors, flea markets and schools!

We are the only country in the world that you can get a pizza at the gym! Thanks Planet Fitness for being part of the problem!

Add to that the stand alone places that specialize in just one thing.
There are **2,800** commercial bakeries and **6,000** retail bakeries in the United States. There are **11,086** Ice Cream Store businesses in the US as of 2022 and there were **37,189** coffeehouse stores nationwide in 2020.

And while there are no hard numbers on stand alone candy shops, I can tell you that we spend <u>3 billion</u> dollars a year on candy for Halloween alone!!! to put that in some perspective according to the American Cancer Society website, donations are about 150 million a year and they have invested around <u>5 billion in research grants since 1946!</u>

You think we got no problem with our priorities?
When a society spends 27 times more money a year on candy for one DAY -then curing cancer....we got problems!
And those number are nothing compared to the 80 billion a year on coffee!

Its no wonder we can not see where healthy food use ends and obsession and addiction begins!

We have 10 times the food stuff then we did just 40 years ago. 10 times more stuff. Like combinations of foods, gums, candy, baked goods, boxed food mixes, prepared foods, frozen foods.
It an obscene and embarrassing orgy of variety.
An embarrassment of riches! Hybrid food, crops and genetically modified foods! We have over 20 artificial sweeteners!
The advancement in "made up foods" and food stuffs over the last 40 years - we are second to none. And one can argue that we have also seen a large rise in health related industries.
Which might seem like one should off set the other.
Has it?

Lets review that:

We have 20 times more Gyms and fitness centers, clubs, classes then we did 40 years an ago.
The home exercise equipment industry is a 6.4 billion a year business.
We have 10 times more health food stores and health food products available at regular stores then ever before in history. An industry worth over 186 billion a year.

The vitamin and supplement industries are hauling in 46 billion on top of that. The global market for alternative medicine and therapies is well over 82 billion a year in value!

And during this time....we have become sicker and sicker. We have developed the absurd competitive epidemics of obesity and malnutrition. And we have reduced the average life expectancy by 3 whole fucking years!!!!!

Which is to say that if you thought that given nothing but better and healthier choices ...we would be healthier?
The numbers do not support that.

And this, more than anything else, is why I have come to the conclusions herein.

**We are not making the right choices.
We are unable to see the compulsions
we are afflicted with.
We are, in fact, food users.
Food abusers.**

And while that is a simple way of saying it, one of the many truths here is that most of what we are "using" is at best bad foods and at worst, not real food at all.

And we are in a constant state of needless consumption.

THREE

Take that out of your mouth!

I have long done mini lectures on the needless consumables. This is a mile long list of things that we simply do not need to live well. And in most cases, these products are not just needless but they are horrible for us and the world we live in.
In a time before this, my wife and I would go to grocery stores and simply marvel at the amount of things that find their way into, not only the store but, your cart. Impostor foods.
Things that we should not eat. And the things that the world would never have had, if anyone would have talked to us about our "little problem" years ago.
These food impostors account for the top ten things sold in grocery stores.
And while they are not the end of the list, they represent a huge amount money, sickness and waste of time and human life.
And on the top of that list is the one thing we are more obsessed about then any other.

Soda.
And I am sorry about this but, this is a completely useless industry that if it fell off the face of the earth tonight while you slept – it would not matter one bit.
And we all would be far healthier for it.

There is no need for this product to exist at all.
There is no benefit and no one can, anywhere, mount a solid argument in favor of soda.
People just drink it.
That's it.
Like its a real and good thing.
Like it is not death in a fucking can!
Feeding our sugar addiction and rotting our bodies from the inside out.

What's incredible is that the average American is drinking about 45 gallons of soda every year. In total that is 375 pounds of that mess pass through your system in 365 days.

Over a pound a day of NOTHING but trouble!

Even crazier is the sugar. 45 gallons totals roughly 470 cans in one calendar year.

A TOTAL OF 20 POUNDS OF CORN SYRUP
A YEAR.
And it is killing us.
Slowly and deliberately.

The soda industry is a 333 billion dollar a
year business in the United States.
The most money spent on soda in the
whole world, is spent here in the USA.

And to put that number in perspective

**We spent a trillion a year in health
insurance in American.
So that soda number is a full 1/3 of
the total money spent on health
insurance!
Another way of putting it is that if we
all stopped buying soda – we could
cover 1/3 of our health insurance
cost!**

And we would also save on total health
costs from the better health we would
enjoy!

Just because ...we like the taste!

Think of it this way.
You walk out back your house every day
and find your neighbor throwing money on
an open fire. When you ask why?

They simply say, because I like the way it looks and smells!
This product should have a label that states: warning this product is
Needless, useless, costly and harmful.
Consume at great risk!

The question is not even why we do it. Its really more, why won't we stop?

There can be no one anywhere in this country by now, like smoking, that does not know that soda is bad for you.
There is no dental condition that is referred to as "milk mouth".
But we got an epidemic of "mountain dew mouth" in areas of the country.

When people consume so much of this poison that it rots their teeth. Where kids drink it before their adult teeth come in!
Toddlers get it in their sip cups!
How is this possible?
Because we like the taste! Duh!

In 1910 there was a doctors study that said that no one should drink more than a bottle of soda a month. Back then those doctors were smoking in the office and even they knew that soda was bad for you in every way!

Plus the obvious things was..why would you drink it at all. It was a drink that was a drug!
The public either does not know or does not remember that Coke was once a drink that contained real Cocaine!
And while it has been suggested that it was a small amount...that's like saying you are only a little pregnant!

Until 1929, the original soda company was getting people hooked on their product with the use of a slight amount of cocaine!
And I tell you this so that you are not confused and maybe think that once the drink was ok for you but now its gone bad!
It was always bad.
And always will be.

Until 1929 they infused the drink with a Schedule II drug and then after they were forced to remove it, they replaced it with caffeine. Slightly less addictive and slightly less of a stimulant in these amounts.
All to make you want more of something that you had no need for.
No use for.
And contained no possible benefit for you.
And was in fact, due to sugar and stimulants, bad for you!

Nothing has changed.
Except they have soda in elementary
schools now!
There are hundreds of these things in our
daily diets. HUNDREDS OF THEM.
These needless consumables.

I like to start with soda because it is a
flash point for the conversations to follow.
And here is why:
you have already started a defence to my
argument. It is happening.
And the reason it is? You are hooked.

Face it, we are not in elementary school
anymore so the argument of "because,
that's why" will not do. It is not an adult
reply to the question of why we do these
things. Eat these things and make
ourselves sick.
   A simple, "I will do whatever I want"
      seems better. A more adult retort.
   However, **under closer examination,
you will see that what you are eating.
What you are craving and the massive
amount of needless crap YOU eat – IS
         NOT WHAT YOU WANT!
   It is what you have been influenced
         and programmed to want.**
And in a sane world.
That should piss you off.
It makes me mad.

You should also know that I am standing
in the biggest empty room in the universe
on this soda issue.
I am all alone in here.
There are a few ancillary causes in the
parking lot of the building this room is in,
like the Minimalist and conservationist, but
even they are not really ready to let the
soda go.
Shit, even Vegans drink soda! Truly, they
are bad vegans but still.
Even my wife. The love of my life. A
natural food consultant, holistic chef, cook
book author and natural living advocate -
does not agree with me on the "nuke the
Coke" plan! And that is frustrating because
the shit is deadly! NO joke!
But the resistance is strong!
And the reason is?
Programming.
Impact and influence from birth.
All known authorities allow it in
moderation.
And, she likes IT!

Recently we moved to Louisville, the
Bourbon capital of the country. We went
to lunch and the server suggested an Old
Fashion cocktail, made with their house
booze and finished with vanilla. The sales
pitch was epic and my wife got one.
She had never had one in her life.

She hated it.
Why?
Not because its poison.
Not because it went against everything she knows to be true and tells others to do.
Nope. She did not like the taste.

And that is why soda and the litany of other needless food impostors win.
Taste.
Taste over health.
Taste over need.
Taste over life.
And most of all, my loving and educated wife believes in the worst of all lies perpetrated on human kind by half witted authorities...
"all things in moderation!"

FOUR

Who is moderating the moderation

Forgive me the slight nod to the graphic
novel, The Watchmen. But really, just who
in the good hell decides what moderation
is?
Where is the chart, graphs or meter? And
just where on the human body is the red
lite that lights up when you've had your
safe limit of shit?

Nowhere!
That where!

The phrase "everything in moderation"
should be removed from the God Dam
language!
Along with other ugly and stupid oxy -
moronic saying.
My favorite other one is
'A little is OK".

Here again, we live in a world where your phone is keeping time based on a feed from a strontium atomic clock at the National Institute of Standards and Technology. Which is so precise that it will neither lose nor gain one second in about 5 billion years of continuous operation.

Yet, you are accepting this nonsensical measurements from the professionals that are in charge of the only life you get!
"A little?"
Just what the hell are we talking about?
No one has a measuring cup wherever these recommendations come from?
And just what is this "a little" suggestion based on?
What science is there that says a "little" consumption of needless and wasteful and dangerous fake food is ok?

Who does such research?
And for what possible sensible reason?
No one!
This is just something people say! Its like saying,
"I ate some and it did not kill me!"

Yet, there it is and you have heard it all your life.
And you have repeated it too.
And this is just one of many stupid concepts competing for the "most dangerous stuff people say to each other" award.

**This absurd notion is based on many a sick thing. Not the least of which is the "treat" theorem.
The dangerous use of food or junk as a reward for something. And this is the road you travel to the hell we are in. The madness that consumes (pun intended) us all.**

The reward system of food is a feedback loop of deadly proportions.

If Moderation is hard to moderate, limiting reward enticements are impossible.

In a world where we are told that we deserve a break today.
That when we are at some fake old world restaurant serving garbage versions of Italian food we are "family".

And where every meal, it would seem, is a precursor to a "treat"... just how are we to walk back this little black hole.

This is the most insidious matrix of all.

An insane and confusing place where eating out is a reward. Then you have a reward at the end of that which is to eat something even worse then the crap you already ate!

Sure, some of this is a hang over from when we were told we could not have any pudding until we eat our meat!
And, a meal out was a treat itself when we were young.
But, with 1 restaurant for every 334 men, women and children in this country?
Clearly, moderation in dining out has sail away too.
We live a reward lifestyle.

We are trained to.
Everybody gets a reward.
Everyone gets a trophy.
And everyone is entitled to desert.
After every meal.
Unless its breakfast, then the treat is the god damn meal!
I mean, if you think that donuts, sugar filled cereals, muffins, danishes, pancakes, french toast, waffles and baked goods are not a treat, your wrong.

And these breakfast things are just a few of the hundreds of things that we never had in abundance in years gone by.

We have foods today as treats that just 80 years ago, you had a hard time finding everywhere.
Ice cream, for instants, was a delicacy. A real honest to goodness treat. You could not get it all the time.
In every store.
In every restaurant.
Everywhere in the country.
And as such, people from that time where not born or raised in that world of free flowing rivers of frozen cream.
Even after the rivers flooded, those people ate the amounts of those treats that they were trained to eat.

My father use to eat an ice cream about every 2 months. If he was still with us, he would be 88 this year. He was not effected by the massive amount of the stuff.
He just followed the patterns of his younger life.
The environmental training of his upbringing.
We do the same thing. The only difference is that now, it is bigger on an order of magnitude then ever in history.

And the narrative of the day, just like the one my father heard, underpins and supports the matrix of the day.

I was at a Kroger in Louisville yesterday and they had 20 doors, 6 shelve high of frozen ice cream buckets, pints, bars and tubs! Plus 5 pallets siting in the walkway to be stocked!

We have one grocery or convenience store for ever 1500 men, women and children in this country! And if your following the math, its staggering.

If we ate ice cream like my father and his contemporaries did. That would be 6 servings per year. Not tubs or pints, servings but, lets just call it an ice cream in general.
6 ice creams per year.

Lets remember that we have 1 store for every 1500 people in the country. And if they all had an ice cream every 2 months that would be 750 ice creams sold per month - per store.
9000 a year per store.

Last thing you need to know is that the average "inventory turns" (the times they sell out everything on the shelves) in grocery is 9-12 a year.

Kroger had 500 facings of ice cream products! And they were 4 to 6 deep per slot! About 4,000 pieces on hand! On a random Tuesday in May!
And their expectations is to then move at least 48,000 units per year. And these units are often multi packs or gallons which provide the buyer 6 – 8 – 12 servings per unit!
Taking the medium at 8 servings. That upwards of 384,000 servings per year per store.
Or, 256 servings each per year – per person.
That's 42 times more then my father use to eat!
You have only two options here.

One, that Kroger, the biggest grocery chain in the country, are fools and buying and throw away ice cream all the time or two, they stock to meet the demand.
If you are a stock holder of Kroger, you know the answer.
Your average Racetrack gas station is holding 300 to 500 pieces on hand. Its everywhere.

Christ, there is a company now that puts mini stores in hotels in the USA. 56,000 hotels and they stock 3 to 5 kinds of ice cream!
And that is by design.
Training requires repetition.
Continuous exposure and purchase reinforcement is also part of the training.
That is why its everywhere.
There is too much money in it to risk you falling away. You must be trained and supported in order for the products to be sold. For you to feed the beast that feeds you.

There can not be in this universe we live in today any such things as moderation. There is nothing close to "a little".
And there can be nothing like a treat "every once in a while".
The reward – treat – consume cycle must be trained and ingrained in your life from the very first day of life.
With the one goal:
Food is no longer a thing of necessity it is happiness, gratification, joy.

And that training comes in all forms.
Some of the most harmful messages come each other.

We take in this feed and then we spit it
out.
Which is not helpful....
Not every addict needs an enabler, but it
sure does help!

FIVE

Talking about food

Because of the pervasive nature of food in our culture, we talk about food a lot.
It is everywhere.
And its no wonder.
We are surrounded by it every minute of every day. And we repeat this information to each other over and over.
Day in and day out.
We will literally be eating a meal and talking about the next one! We will call people or text them about a new place to eat. Like its a new theme park that opened!
We talk, talk, talk about food in a way that once you stop doing it – it will seem like a compulsion when you hear others doing it.
I wish it was not true but, it is.

Food is no longer a meal or a thing we do three times a day to live.
It is an event.
Entertainment.
A hobby.
A lifestyle. And anthropologist will tell you this is because we spent most of our developing tens of thousands of years looking for it. But today?

We come by this dishonestly.

The advertising and narratives about food stem from a mega industry of unbelievable size and scope. The money spent on this collection of hundreds of industries is more than the GDP of about 50 countries!
The massive amount of things surrounding food is impossible to list but, some of those number have to be talked about.
Take a look at these numbers:

Food content is exploding on YouTube and generates nearly 41 billion views a month!

According to a study conducted by Millward Brown Digital, Firefly, and Google in 2014, nearly half of all adults watch food videos on YouTube

**And according to Google
Almost 30% of the 5 billion videos that are watched on You tube every single day are food related.
Which means we are watching
1.66 billion videos a day about food**

The food network latest line up boast over 500 food shows!! on one channel!

And couple hundred on Netflix, Hulu and others.

Roughly 17.8 million cookbooks were sold in the United States in 2018

We had 6.9 billion dollars worth the meal kits delivered to our doors in 2021

The Cooking class industry is worth 2 billion a year from over 1250 business employing over 15,000 people.
The global culinary tourism market reached a value of US$696.5 Billion in 2021. And is expected to double by 2027. because it is not enough to eat and talk and live for food...we have to travel and eat and talk about that food somewhere else...

Food, beverage and restaurant companies spend almost $14 billion per year on advertising in the United States:
That is almost twice the drug companies spend a year!!!!
and
Twice what is spent on AIDS worldwide each year!
We spend 616 billion a year at convenience stores in the US.
Compared that to medical research yearly.

The NIH invests about $41.7 billion annually in medical research for the American people.

41.7 billion is 1/12 of the money spent on bad snacks and roller food!
These number tell a story so insane it is not possible to explain. That one type of crap filled store gets that much money while, research is less than 1/12 of that.

Its the equivalent of your local bank only having a sign that says "beware of dog" as protection! And not even really having a dog...just the sign!

The statistic shows The U.S. food storage container market was valued at around 475 million U.S. dollars in 2016, and was forecast to reach about 570 million dollars by 2021. that money is staggering – just to store the shit!

The home appliance industry, which includes electrical or mechanical devices used in a household, is a multi-billion dollar industry.

The global retail sales of major and small appliances amounting to more than 420 billion U.S. dollars in 2020.

**It is estimated that the total number of world recipes is 5 trillion and that is more recipes then there are atoms in the universe!
But there is nothing wrong here!
Everything is fine.**

The input is all encompassing.
There are hundreds of food, cooking and recipe magazines.

Even the Bible refers to food 1,207 times!

There is no where to hide from the programming that surrounds food.

And even if there was, would we be self aware enough to realize we were addicted?

All the evidence says no.

FOOD SICK NATION

SIX

It can't get any worse!

Yes, it can.
I know that somewhere in your head there
is a thought.
A hope.
That there is some small silver lining to
this whole thing. Or, at least, it can't get
any worse. But, it can.
And, it does.

Because there is another narrative out
there that is even more corrosive to health
and the human condition. And that
narrative comes from all of this
programming that most people do not
even know is effecting them.
And that point can not be overstated.
If you did not know this before this
reading, then be very worried about the
information and guidance you get from
professionals that are as unaware as you
were 46 pages ago.

This goes far beyond the "moderation" advice.
It almost criminal.
Research and studies are skewed.
How could they not be?
They are starting from a place that is not based in what one might call a "base reality".

And let me be clear here. If you are thinking that a little of something is OK. And that is the conventional wisdom of the times. Then your deductions and conclusions are going to be slightly off target.
This might be confusing for you so lets do this first.

A primer on bad thought:

We view life on this planet as fleeting. Any human lifespan is but a blip on the timeline of the universe.
This narrative is pervasive.
This has lead us to incorporate some very poor ideas on how we should spend our time here.
One of these poor ideas is the notion that since we have only this one life and its so short – why deny ourselves of anything.

Another is an augmented version of that,
which is the moderate idea.

Next we have the "YOLO" concept.
You only live once.
And as such, you should do whatever and
enjoy it all.

These are all sprung from the same womb
and they all lead to the mess we have
today.
And the way we think about food and the
way we do not think about food.

However, there is another narrative. One
that has come from a very limited view,
and it is used to underpin the other word
path.
This view is based on only observational
research (the oldest and least scientific).

It states that we have been eating these
things (the Standard American Diet -SAD)
for a few hundred years and we are still
living longer than before.

It claims, without any proof at all, that
frozen food is just as good as fresh.
It says that GMO is no different than
heirloom crops.

And that chemical alteration and preservatives and anything else we can think up in Frankenstein's lab to do to food – simply does not matter because the human body will keep on working.

And it is this kind of thinking – bad thinking that has lead doctors to claim that vitamins do not work.
Or do not help and that you can get everything from food without even knowing that they are talking about food that is no longer food as nature intended!

All the while facing a tidal-wave of sickness and epidemic numbers of preventable disorders!
They do not know because they are unaware that the influences that have lied to you – not only lied to them but it has drilled its way deep into the minds that should be able to remove preconceived notions and let research go were ever it goes.
Thus, their conclusions will be skewed!

How else can you explain a group of people that believe competing narratives.
One that the body can cope with anything and the other that everybody breaks down and gets sick.

When nigher are necessarily true. But, most of them are indeed connected.

They blissfully tell people that the body can take a lot and that it will compensate and that we are hard to kill. And its insane to worry about every little thing you put in your body and that we all should just get on with our lives.
And that is all based on bad thinking!

Its a form of mass destruction. A huge pile of conformation bias. Where you look for things that only support your point of view. In this case the flimsy notion that if it has not killed us – it will not.

And that has lead them to do other kinds of awful things.
Like raise the bar for how many side effects we should allow from medication.
Reduce our concern for long term effects.
Tell people that a little will not hurt you. And in general give bad, slanted and ill advised advice.

A better way of putting it might be that they live in a world where they expect you to be sick.
To hurt.

To poison yourself and that you will not do
the right thing anyhow.
Then they give you pills that will kill you in
a different way and tell you that's helpful.

All because they do not know what the
right thing is to begin with.
Look I know that you might think I'm
being to harsh on the medical community

but I have had them argue with me, with
the same passion <u>against healthy eat</u> and
<u>for the use of drugs!</u>
Like an insane person might.
I have seen them tell me that it doesn't
matter what you eat. Then tell everyone
they see that they are all pre diabetic!

Confidently assure their customers that
they will die of something and that
everything is OK in moderation!

Why would they do this?
Its not because they are evil.
They are not working for some
madman in some hollowed - out
volcano layer!
No, they are ill informed and unaware
of the truth. The truth that should be
so easy to see.

You are what you eat!

But how can something so simple and non sexy compete against the wall of media and influence.

Gain any ground in the race with trillions of dollars at play in the markets of death and body destruction!

How can anyone make a case for not trading off our health for a quick high in a world where no one will tell us the truth and most of them don't know it anyhow.

Just like the reward cycle, we trade off a few minutes of bliss from bad food for hours of pain and years of suffering and then have another group of enablers tell us we would have died from something anyhow!

And if you can not see where that kind of thinking will lead, you have not been paying attention.
The true cost of these denial and deceit is not just your liver or kidneys.

It is not paid only with human suffering around the world.

Because this same kind of cavalier attitude towards our health and food and chemicals and pursuit of pleasure over reason has let people justify the poisoning of the ground and water and air.
The planet can take it and it will not matter what we do, the world will end someday anyhow and we will not be alive to see it.
These insane, nihilistic notions are pervasive in our society.
Its not just about our sick addiction to food.
Our insane dysfunctional relationship with food and eating. It has spilled over into how we treat each other and the planet.

It is one of the major reasons our world is an environmental nightmare.
These foods we do not need are resource hogs, pollutant orgies and world killers!

And because if this programmed bad thinking, they even have more insane and dangerous ideas on "fixing" the problem.

So yeah, it does get worse.

SEVEN

Useless Industries are environmental apex predators!

A few chapters a go, I took some shots at soda. From a pure and simple -its a killer point of view. However, we need to return to the fountain again.

I know that it is not a popular notion that the fake food and useless food industries are the cause of environmental woes but ....its true.
And unlike all the rules and laws and regulations needed to stop dumping, burning fossil fuels and promoting alternative energy before we melt the polar caps....

You and I can fix this part of the problem.
We can start today.
However, the powers that be. Those bad
thinkers. They have a few bad ideas of
their own. And they all come from the
same ignorance.

So lets review this issue:
Our world is getting hotter every day.
The climate is changing,
ancient ice is melting and we face
simultaneous epidemics
of droughts and flooding.
Unprecedented storms and forest fires
Summers of scorching heat and winters of
arctic cold.

We protest and demand green energy
and for some better science to save us
and beg for the powers that be to listen
and change!
To stop polluting.
Stop clear cutting our forests and
burning the land
Making millions of gas powered pollution
devices every year.

in short
we want everything that is out of our
control to fix the problem.
We blame everyone else.

And want the same people that let the
mess happen – to fix it.

Do you know who is behind green energy?
companies like;
Georgia pacific
GE
Shell oil
BP
and they are working on this problem for
you?

You know what can happen when you just
relax and let politicians, wall street,
oil companies and big business
fix anything?

They just might work in their interest and
not yours

**Their interest is in keeping things the
way they are and to that end
they have denied climate change,
lied about their practices and lobbied
to keep oil, gas, coal, fracking,
nuclear and every other thing they
have trillions of dollars invested in it
and profit from it.**

These people are running on the same bad
software as everyone else. And they really
believe that everyone will die anyhow...so
much so that they have started to warm
up to a new and terrifying idea for a one
time big fix

And this idea is coming from top minds in
the field.
Get rid of people!
The most recent research says that one
sure fire way to help heal the planet is
reduce the population!

This idea is gaining ground.
The website www.populationmatters.org is
all about it. They are saying, without a
shred of backup, that we should institute
mandatory population control!
Because nothing else will work!

Which should come as some surprise to
the people of Thailand in a recent article it
states simply that forced reduction in
births has made no difference.

Even still, this insane though process
which is no different than the one that lets
us eat trash and die young, has a new and
even more stupid idea!
that's right, you got to go!

**Even though you and all your friends
do not run an oil refinery or pipeline.
No one you know makes government
energy policy and you have never
tossed a bag of trash in the ocean.
Or burned the woods
or clear cut a rain forest!**

You are the problem!

There are just too dam many of you pesky
people.
and if there were less of you..
We could just all keep doing what we do.
Burning, drilling, using and wasting and
everything would be fine.

Like an engineered version on the rapture!
And just who would get to decide which of
us could have children?
And what's next?
Would we stop feeding impoverish parts of
the world?
Ignore the needs of the many for the good
of the few?
or maybe we just go Hollywood and start
up the purge!
This is what you get from starting off with
bad thinking!
Wrong thinking.
Fatalistic, nothing can be fixed, everything
breaks thinking!

Yet, another idea is out there too, to confuse you even more and muddy the waters.
A growing group of people say we can do something right now to help this problem.
And they are using our environmental nightmare to underpin their agenda of a totally plant based diet.
They want us to stop farming for livestock and that will save us from total destruction.
Because cows belch and fart methane and they eat and drink too damn much!
Not kidding!
In this interesting universe they see us farming too much to feed livestock.
So we would stop that.
And then we would eat only plant based foods.
Which we would grow, I guess, where we use to grow feed for the cows?

Now no one is asking where the livestock goes when we stop eating them.
and its a fair question.

Currently, we have a combined total of chickens (19 billion), cows (1.5 billion), sheep (1 billion) and pigs (1 billion) living at any one time.

Presumably these would all be set free
from their bondage and let loose to live
free range for the rest of their days in
bliss!

Yeah, about that...
you need
1.8 ac for each cow or 2.7 billion ac for
them to be free and not eat feed
10 sq. ft per chicken
or 3.8 million ac

250 sq. ft. per pig
or 5.8 million ac.

and a staggering
½ ac per lamb
or 500 million ac for them eat free.

Adding up to
3.2 billion acres of free range grazing land
needed to support these animals until
their death.
There is only 4.6 billion acres of crop land
in the world right now!

So if we all just stop eating them and ate
their food instead. We would need all of
their crop land and then we would have to
relocate them somewhere ...
3.2 billion acres of somewhere!

If they were to just take over the lower 48 that would only be about 1.9 billion acres. and they would also need all of central America about half of South America too!

Unless we were gong to just kill them at once or eat them till their were gone?
I'm guessing not...

It's funny that these two ideas mirror the "Doctors vs Health food nuts" in their position and poorly thought out ideas that are based only in what they believe or want.

Not on real facts or scientific truths.

I'm not kidding here...they have no plan
But what if both crazy camps are half right?
We need to reduce, but not people and not animals!
What if we could all be healthier, clean the air and water. Reduce carbon out put by half and reduce pollution by 75%
And what if we could do this with no new technologies or green energy production?

I know there is nothing less sexy then
simple common sense reduction of food
that we do not need.
but….
it is the key to saving this whole thing.

And it is literally those thousands of things
you can put in your body that are not
needed for our existence.
That are also bad for us and the planet.

But…are there industries out there that
are bigger then meat that we could get rid
of without suffering any nutritional issues?
YES
And so, We have to go back to the
fountain.
The first set of things that have zero use
in the body and it is just a few contents of
soda.
Because they are sugar & corn crop heavy

They are supported by a massive amount
of fuel needed for transportation and are
all in cans or plastic bottles made from
petroleum that are filling land fills and we
have plastics now in our bodies:

Lets start with the completely useless
drink industry:

237. billion in soda a year world wide

85 million in energy drinks
675 billion in dairy milk sales
23. billion non dairy milk products

Meat is a 900 billion world wide industry:
the 4 needless drink markets above are
over 1 trillion plus alone.
(note that: 675 billion is from dairy milk
which is a totally useless drink that no one
needs unless you are a baby cow)

These industries are producing
400 billion plastic bottles a year and some
one, somewhere is worried about cows
and pigs?

And as far as reducing feed crops..
milk cows represent 1/3 of the cow
population and live up to twice as long as
beef cows.
so they are fed twice as long.
by eliminating milk from our diets, we
could remove over 60% of the farm to
feed issue!

This would also remove huge tanker
trunks filled with MILLIONS of gallons of
milk from the highway. Reducing co2,
reducing oil use, heat and water use.

And this is not a thing we need to run by
congress.

We just stop drinking this crap that is useless and needless and harming us and the planet.

If your really serous about saving your life and the planet, we could just go ahead and tank the coffee market. Coffee is 100 billion world wide market.
And it doesn't grow everywhere. Add on fuel from the shipping via land, sea and air. The Co2 in processing and roasting and the support industries like cups and lids.
Think the cups and lids don't matter? According to the Starbucks's facebook post from January 2017, they sold 671 million cups of coffee in 2016. They are just one company! And they are pushing out hundreds of millions of paper cups and plastic lids a year!
Starbucks uses 800 million pounds of coffee a year. That's only 5% of the total use a year.
Which means we farm, roast, transport, drip and drink 16 billion pounds of coffee a year!
16 billion pounds of a crop that is totally worthless to your health.

Bad for the planet and the peripheral waste and energy use is hurting the environment.

I could go on and on, but the point of this
exercise is to understand that what is bad
for your body is also bad for your planet.
That bad thinking and living unaware of
the facts and truths has caused us to be
poor shepherds of our selves and the
earth.
That the consequence of our addictions do
not stop with us. We are not the only
victims.
That our addiction is kill both us and the
planet..
And, lastly, by eliminating them, we save
both.

So, yeah
We got a problem with food.

How we think and use and grow and eat
and burn and dump and waste and ignore
and pass the responsibility.

We got problems.

And like everything else, knowing there is
a problem is the first step to solving it.

Yet, no addict can start recovery when
they are in denial and everyone is in a
constant state of denial.

EIGHT

The attitude of denial

There is an attitude of denial that is common in our health and our world. This cavalier attitude is that nothing is going to hurt us.
That nothing will hurt the planet.
That we simple and small humans could not possibly cause any harm to this giant blue orb.

You have heard this from people all around you.
You tell them that smoking us bad for them and they tell you that everyone dies from something.
You say that cars pollute the air and they call you a snowflake. Or a tree hugger.
You say that global warming is changing the climate, and they say there is no such thing.

Or it's a cycle that happens every few million years that we have nothing to do with.

The only problem with all of these denials is... the are based on NOTHING... not one God dam fact.
The facts are that in the last 150 years, humans have advanced and populated across this planet in a way that has never happened in the history of the world.

Things that have never happened have no historical data to use to demise them as safe or harmless.
And I am not talking about using a new kind of dish soap.

These changes and new things are mind-blowing and huge. Massive changes and advancements have resurfaced the world. Take pollution:

150 years ago, there was no human-made pollution in the air. Today, it's a mess up there.

We have detonated over 2000 nuclear bombs in the past 70 years. Just testing them! Not including the ones we dropped in Japan.

We have had 4 nuclear power planet disasters since 1961. Spilling massive amounts of nuclear pollution into the atmosphere.

We have about 1.44 billion cars in the world as of 2022. Spewing pollution into the air every minute of every day.

23 million big rigs and commercial trucks on the roads worldwide.

We have over 40 million planes flights a year around the world.

We have launched over 70 thousand rockets into the atmosphere and into space!!!! In the past 70 years.

350,000 trains in the world. 95 % are diesel.

We have designed and have in use 350,000 chemicals for commercial use every day.

We have drilled and abandoned over 29 million oil wells in the past 120 years. And currently have 1.5 million in use.

There are 2400 coal burning power planets worldwide. Running 24 hours a day.

We have paved 33 billion meters of roads,
which is around 4 million miles of
blacktop!

We cut down 15 billion trees a year.

You take a good look at that list.
It is not a full list, just the highlights.

And tell me we have not had an impact on
the world.
And none of these things ever happened a
hundred years ago.

Yet, these denial assholes will tell you that
none of this will hurt the planet or you.
Just like the people who say that bad food
and fake food can't hurt them.

This ignorance is staggering and
dangerous.
And without any proof.

There is simply no way to know how much
damage these things have caused.

And do not let them tell you that they
know because you can't know a thing that
has never happened before.

A good rule of thumb would be this. If you would not want it in your house or on your lawn or in your drinking water at home.. then we probably should do it anywhere.

But we have this belief that we are separate from the world and its systems. That we can protect ourselves and pollution the planet and keep those things apart. It's not just silly. It's completely insane.

You would not run a car inside your house. Even if you survived the flames, the stains and damage to the inside of your home would be intense.
You would not want radioactive materials in your kitchen or bedroom or your babies room. So why would you be ok with it in the air. The water. The world.

Everything is connected. There is no separation between you and your world. And the sooner we can accept that, the better off this world and your health will be.

The truth is that even if there is no global warming, these practices are wrong.
This way of thinking and acting is wrong.
Dumping pollution into the water, air, and ground is wrong.

It's the wrong thing to do.
Even if it never had an environmental impact, it is not how people are supposed to act.
You don't throw trash on your lawn or your neighbors lawn. You just don't do it.

You do not live in filth or act without thinking or concern for others. And of course, these things are harmful and we all know it.
When it comes to how these acts harm the environment, we do know what can happen.

Not included in the long list a few pagers ago is the 1300 EPA super fund sites around the USA that are so toxic and contaminated that we hardly even know how to mitigate the damage.
There are tire fires that have been burning for 4 decades.

And there are sites like the old St. Louis Airport site that was a dumping ground for a Manhattan project research facility that has an underground fire of nuclear contamination solid that is an unimaginable danger. Nothing I can think of this more terrifying then that! They can not put it out – they have no idea how to!

People do not even want to acknowledge these things exist.
To do so is to admit we have data on the effects of bad practices.

We justify what we do or do not do with the worst of all lies.
The one that says whatever comes from our neglect and negligence will happen long after the current " we" are dead. As if we have no responsibility to our future fellow humans.

This denial, avoidance, and justifications only deny us our collective future. It serves no purpose to pretend that you know something that you don't. It just makes you look foolish.

But, like the addiction and sick relationship we have with food. We have this inability to see that we should make healthy, safe practices a priority. As high a priority as our personal health and money.

But who shows us this?
From government leaders to our new billionaires, just who is leading this charge?
Showing us that this matters?

Teaching us that you can be successful
and rich and exercise good stewardship of
this world and ourselves?

Name that person!
The 3 richest men in this world are
actively spending money on and getting
attention for their efforts to build in space
and colonize other planets!

They are not using their unprecedented
wealth to clean up this world.
Fix these problems.
Feed the hungry or cure the sick.

No, they are looking elsewhere for a fresh
start.
And even though they do not come out
and say it, their actions seem to suggest
that they could care less what happens
here.
Or worse, they think that these problems
can not be solved.

Messages, training, environmental impact.
Social cues and outright narratives driven
by skewed priorities have shaped our
collective view of this world and ourselves.
Our place here.
Our relationship and responsibility to this
world.

Put us in a place in our minds and hearts
that point directly to a simple and
debilitating notion that we are small,
helpless and unable to change or fix or
effect anything on this earth or in our own
bodies.
That we should just enjoy this short life.
Live only for today and feel no
responsibility for anything or anyone that
follows.

It is a destructive contradictory
thought pattern.
We feel helpless and weak.
We are convinced we are only one person
and can change nothing. So we live only
for ourselves.
Yet that very behavior is the thing that
keeps us from trying to fix anything.
Change anything.
And if we never try to stop.
To control ourselves.
To demand change.
Then we never have any proof we can
affect this world or our health.
Then we can feel confident in just doing
whatever we want.
Living as selfish and unaware as we want
to.
Tossing out those lies and justification
when someone confronts us and then
making fun of those willing to try.

Calling them fools.

It is a self reinforcing delusion.
A story we tell ourselves that is separate
from reality and fact.
One that is a closed loop.
The actions we take create the outcome.
And the outcome is used to excuse the
actions we take.

NINE

ME FIRST

This attitude is not new.
It has been around a very long time.

Winston Churchill is credited with saying;

"If you are young and not a liberal, you have no heart. If you are old and not a conservative, you have no sense. "

This sentiment is echoed in all things in our society today. It is another cornerstone of these narratives that have confused us.

If you think about it. The older a person gets, the more they see.
And learn.
Then they would be the ones worried about what they would be leaving for the next generations.
They would have the knowledge and history to draw on to see what has been done wrong.

But no, not in our society. Our society and this statement is a cornerstone of this Me First mentality.

What he really meant was that young people do not know enough to realize they can change nothing. But they have the time to waste thinking about others in the world.
But the older you get, you better stop that and only work to security your personal future and wealth.

Promoting the notion that older people should care less about this world and the right things. And act only in their self-interest.

It is a contradictory matrix because this "me first" really is only about money and security. And from this comes the choices of cheap, useless empty food looking things that will fill you up but feed you nothing.
Indulgences and treats you need from the sacrifices you make to earn a living.

The quick fixes of sweets and even the use of drugs that let us "escape" are all used to counter this inexplicably socially amoral society we live in.

One where you can never seem to earn enough. Own anything. Figure out its system.
Always wanting.
Always under the gun. While the goals and security we need are forever being pushed further and further away.

Why wouldn't people simply give up.
Go for themselves.
Eat and do whatever they want.
Find escape and reward where ever they can.

Its not excusing our complicity in it. Its not blaming society for our choices. But to say that this system and its trappings are not part of the problem would be a lie.

The basic "me first" attitude has grown out of all this. And its effect on our health, our minds and our planet are everywhere.

There have been many iterations of this notion over the years. And the lack of security for every one has played a part in people turning inward and only working in their own best interests.

Many an event over the last 60 years have helped us get to this point in history.
Market crashes.

Recessions, wars, acts of terror. The changes in how and where and for how much we work.
Designer foods and crap on the cheap offered to make your 12 hour work and commute day easier.
All of these things have pushed the average person off balance. Made them feel stressed and taken so much of their time and effort to overcome, they simply can not think of others even if they wanted to. They cant stop to eat right. Buy good food and cook at home.

Which is to say that not all selfish acts are from really selfish people. And the "me first" is not the same as being a genuine selfish person.

Yet, even thought all if this is part of it, no one but you can start to change things.

As a counter to Churchill's quote, I often think of this one by Gandhi;

"be the change you want to see in the world".

And we come to the point where we understand the how and why and details of the system that underpins this "user" world.

The forces that push us towards
dependency and addiction and selfish
destructive behaviors.

The programming and environmental
impacts that have been here from our first
breath.
The juggernaut of billion dollar businesses
that need you to not care about yourself
or your world in order for them to profit.

We accept these things.

And then, we have to push them aside and
begin to act in a way that will save us and
in turn save our world.

We now come to the part of the plan that
is always the hardest.

The part were we have to do something.
And its a big thing now.

Because you are not just choosing to
change for yourself.
Or your loved ones.

I would hope that, by now, you can see
that the choice to change is for a higher
propose.

For the longevity of you and our planet.

You are no longer able to think that the choices that you make have no effect on anyone but you.

And that should make you feel good. That when you stop the buying and consuming of needless wasteful harmful products, you will help your body and you are joining a group of people that are literally being an active part of the solution.

Now, will this knowledge overcome personal and psychological reason you might have with your food addiction?
No.

And as I said in the beginning of the book, these problems can not just be solved by any book.

However, for those that take the first steps towards freedom, this one reason can be something to hold on too.

And when it comes to change, we can all use more reasons to stay the course than we have for continuing to make poor choices.

That said.

If your ready to help yourself and our planet.

We are going to need to detox the life you lead.
Not just the food you eat.

FOOD SICK NATION

TEN

Behavioral Detox

When we want to change our lives, we need fresh and new surroundings and habits as much as we need fresh and natural foods.
This does not mean you have to go to meetings or move to the Himalayas. There are some basic things that you can do to help you change how you think of about and relate to food.

Thinking of food as fuel is a good place to start.
Thinking of food as something you get from your home is another.

Basic things to help change the cycles we are in.

The unconscious habits of add ons, extras, treats, snacks and sweets.

The addition of some basic things we all need to live.

And removing temptation and social pressure by avoidance.

There are 3 behavioral Detox rules to start, each can help you on the path to freedom.

And Doing these 3 things for a few weeks - can yield some startling results.

People often have more energy, sleep better and begin to see the world in a different way.

There is a lot that goes into kicking any habit and these things are often talked about more than the feeling of satisfaction you get from being free.

Of not being dragged around by your cravings and dependencies.

The feel of knowing that you are in charge.
You have taken back some control.

DETOX rule #1

Avoid media, menus and manipulation.

As a former smoker, I can tell you that while there are no cigarette ads on TV anymore, people still smoke in the movies, and short format streaming shows, AKA series.
And it was troubling for me to watch in the beginning.
However, the advertising for food, eating, restaurants and cooking is an avalanche every 10 minutes on network broadcast TV.
Stop watching Network TV, just for a week or two. And no cooking shows. Watch movies or just go out and do something else.
Take up a forgotten hobby.
Occupy your mind with other things.
Remember the day you were too busy to eat?
You did not die.
I'm not saying to starve, I'm only making the point that if you are thinking about other things.
Your less likely to obsess over food.

**We have to own the truth that we
need 3 - 20 minute time slots to fuel
up the body. Think of your car. It has
no tastes for Exxon or BP, it just
needs gas.
Food is fuel.
Nothing more.
It's the stuff that lets you be able to
live your life – it is not YOUR LIFE!**

You have never had a friend come back
from vacation and show you pictures of all
the gas stations they stopped at.
Its the stuff in between those fill ups - that
was the trip!

When you see an ad for food, crap or
soda, remember the multi trillion dollar
industries that are behind it.

Remember that they want and need you
to fail. To quit your quest to save all of us
and just feed them.
Consider this;
if you had a friend that was an alcoholic.
Would you invite him over and place full
glasses of his favorite drink on every
table?
Would you gulp down tall cold glasses of
booze in front of him while smiling and
letting out sounds of orgasmic pleasure
with each sip?

Would you entice him with coupons that
he could use to get their drug or drink of
choice at a lesser cost?
Or have some swimsuit model half naked
inviting him to join her in a binge?
No, you know he has a problem and its
killing him. That kind of behavior is like
the stuff that demons would do!

Well….. that what they are doing.
They not only know you have a problem –
their whole fucking business model is
based on your willingness to kill yourself
slowly. You smarten up – they go out of
business!

Think of them as merchants of death! That
should stall your automatic response to
buy and eat.
Consider it as a primal issue. Its them or
you! They got to go!

Lastly, if you do have to eat somewhere
other than your own kitchen.
Read the menu.
Not for yummy meals. Look for food that
you might be able to make at home from
scratch.
Stick to plain chicken and vegetables.
You'll notice that on these menus, the
healthier choices are also the cheaper
ones! Less nonsense.

They are not covered or smothered or contain 12 other ingredients.

Another good rule for eating out is to choice the meal that looks like it will not be enough for you. We are trained by time to indulge in restaurants.

Over indulge. If you think about it, when was the last time you left one of these death pit-stops and felt that you had "just enough"?

The menu is designed to get you to buy more.
They entice you with add on things at a value price.
They show bigger pictures of the appetizers and desserts because you came there to eat a main course.
Its the menu and the servers job to sell you more. Up sell you on drinks, sides, sauces, starters and more.

Like a dealer asking you if you'd like some heroin with that bag of weed. Or a new pipe or bong? Or a fresh pack of clean needles!
These places should be seen as demonic pusher dens.

Because they are.

Lastly, avoid group eating.
It is always about meeting up somewhere.
Just say your busy.

You can't be in social eating situations for
a while until you have a better understand
of how to control them.

FOOD SICK NATION

DETOX rule #2

D.I.Y.

Best practice in the first few weeks is to be in complete charge of what goes in your food before it goes in your body...which means to cook it yourself.
This may be the hardest thing to do.

Recent numbers show that we are cooking less and less.
Only 46% of Americans says they cook from 5 to 7 nights a week.

29% of people cook three to four nights a week. That's 98 million people

12% cook one or two nights.
That's 40 million people.

7% do it less often than once a week.
That's 23 million people

3% never cook at home.

(3% also said they "don't know" how often they cook dinner.)
That's over 20 million people eating every meal out of the house.

Now, you might have already seen this from those numbers but, they say nothing about breakfast and lunch.

And there is a good reason for that. Because only 35% of Americans eat breakfast every day at all!

21% have it 4-6 days a weekend

20% have it 1-3 days a weekends

12% a few times a MONTH

6% a few times a YEAR

6% simply do not eat breakfast ever!
And no one seems to make or cook it for themselves.
And for lunch, it is all out of the house.

On average, Americans spend 2500.00 a year on work day lunches.

You could pay for your cell phone and 9 of the top streaming channels a year with that money!

In total, The average American individually
spends $1,200 a year on fast food alone,
while the average American household
spends around 10% of their income.
That adds up to $110 billion dollars a year,
which could end world hunger for up to
three years.

Even when people are "making a meal"
they are using prepared foods. Frozen
foods.
Meal kits and manufactured food stuffs
rather than using fresh meats and
vegetables.
So those at home cooking numbers are
really lower if you were to weed out the
fresh food meals from the rest.

In general, flushing out the crap begins
with the understanding that 90% of what
you eat is not food or necessary for life.
And if it is not necessary then it is an
indulgence!

All of these meals out of your own kitchen
or per-manufactured for you to heat and
eat are loaded with bad fats, hidden
sugars, extra sodium from all kinds of
sources, chemicals and additives and
things to preserve colors and texture and
freshness.

Many of these things are addictive. Sugar
and sodium make you crave more of the
same.
Things like MSG not only alter your brain
chemistry but they change you taste bubs,
causing a swelling of the your taste
sensors to make you think it taste better.

It's the culinary version of getting high
and finding things funny.
Its not the entertainment that's better –
it's your perceptions that are skewed !

You find these substances in prepared
foods, can foods, boxed foods, shelf stable
foods, frozen meals, dressing, sauces,
powdered cheese mixes, cheap ice cream,
ground meats like pork sausage, breakfast
sausage, packaged and deli sliced lunch
meats.

All of it designed to get you hooked and
keep you coming back for more more
more!

Remember, we want to eat food.
We just do not want to _use_ food.
So keep it simply.
And keep it in YOUR KITCHEN.

DETOX rule #3

Water, water, water

Diets, in general, have a nasty habit of telling you to remove stuff from your plate but never give you any replacement for them. Leaving you with less choices and a sense that you will never be full again.

So, before you start cutting out bad foods and snacks and fast food crap, you need to do a full week on something you need anyhow.
Water!

This is not a water fast – you just add in the water to your normal diet!

Drinking water has become a real problem in our land. Mainly due to the massive load of "drinks" out there. There is nothing found in nature, that is ready to drink in it's natural state but water.
Every thing else you need some process to drink.

Sure you can drink coconut milk but you need to break it open first. Yes, you can juice fruit, but again – that's a process too.
Humans need pure water. And a lot of it! 3 oz of water every half hour (of waking hours).
Not 8 – 8oz glasses. Or chugging 32 oz at a time.

Just a habit of drinking small amounts all day will get you hydrated without bloating you. And over the course of 16 hours, at 3 oz each, you will get close to 96 oz in.

Studies have shown that often people mistake thirst for hunger.

So, if you are not sure – drink a small amount of water and wait a beat.

The water thing has been beaten to death as advice goes.
So just know you need it and do it in these small and consistent doses.

You will notice by the end of the first week that you have drank less soda, coffee, tea and whatever else you normally poison yourself with.

As the days goes on, you will crave water!
It is the best craving you'll ever have. You
will also start to really notice how many
people never drink water!

Do not let anyone tell you that we do not
need water. Or that water is in a lot of
drinks. These are half truths and out right
lies.
Pure water is the only thing we need to
drink.
Everything else is man made.

ELEVEN

WHAT TO EAT

Once you have a few weeks on the
behavioral detox, you can start changing
out foods you eat for real human food.

There is nothing more upsetting to me in
this whole wide world than the knowledge
that most people do not know what
humans are supposed to eat.

And before you say they do know....
Consider this;
Real human food is not complicated to
explain – its just hard to accept.

And because of that, even the people that
know – don't say too much about it.

**In the simplest of terms, human food
is food that is found in its natural
form. Then it is
picked off a plant or tree or hunted
down and killed.**

See, easy to explain.

Now go to your kitchen and start looking for it.
And remember that if it is frozen – that's not in its natural form.
Dehydrated or preserved in cans or boxes? Not natural form.

Now since we do not all have farms, we will need to suffer some refrigeration but other than that?
Keeping it fresh and natural is the rule.
As far as shopping;
Your time there will be short, since you no longer need to walk up and down every lane of the store. Grabbing up boxes and bags of dry good. No baked goods or deli meats or sodas.
No more grocery safari for you.

When you shop for your new food, you will be spending the bulk of your time in the produce section and then the meat sections where you will be buying salad stuffs, fresh green vegetables, some potatoes or yams, fresh meat and seafood.
Stopping quickly by the dairy section to get all natural eggs and some real "live' cheese – no American cheese, that's not real. You will also need some natural balsamic vinegar and real olive oil for salad dressing.

And then?
Out the doors!
You should pay first...I guess, but then
you are heading home to cook!
Where you will be making 2 plates of food
3 times a day.

As follows:
A large green salad on one full plate with a
natural, non creamy, full fat dressing.
¼ of the other plate will be protein, which
should be lean beef, fish or eggs.
(Chicken and turkey are lesser proteins
but, OK in a pinch) and the rest of that
plate will be streamed green vegetables.
3 times a day.

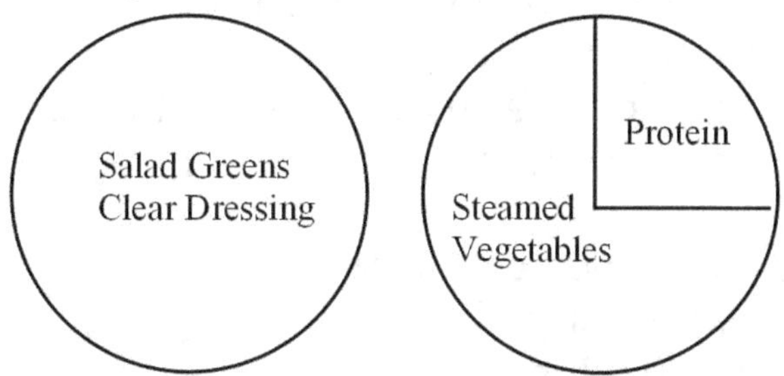

Yes, even at breakfast!
No, no toast!

Now here's the thing.
You are going to say things to yourself
here like

"I can't eat that" or "how can I get by on that?"
That is just the addiction talking.
Looking for reasons why this is impossible.

There is nothing impossible about eating real natural human foods.

It is just not what you are use to or what the multi billion dollar food industries want you to do.
There will be people that say this is not true.
That we have been eating grains and bread and milk and whatever for thousands of years.
And that's true.
Yet, humans have been here for hundreds of thousands of years.
These things are the real human food.
And I can prove it. It is not complicated.

In the absence of the simplest forms of food processing like; Cooking, grinding, milling, soaking etc.
What could a human eat on this big blue world?
Because, without any of our cool processes – we would be eating things...raw!

I am not saying to eat raw meat, I am only saying that if it is consumable in its natural raw form – then it follows that it is human food.

That list would be easy to write and include: beef, fish, lamb, eggs, nuts, seeds, vegetables and fruits.

Any meat that you could order rare, is a natural human food.

Any plant you can eat without any form of cooking is natural human food.

Anything you can find to drink in nature... water, is what humans need.

Things we must have well done like chicken, pork, bottom feeder seafood like shrimp and lobster, crab, scallops etc are not natural human foods.

Roots and tubers that need to be cooked or soaked are not natural human food.

Grains need to be ground, soaked or cooked in order for us to digest them – they are not natural human foods.

Even dried fruit is a process and in that process, we decrease the water contain of the fruit and increase the sugar content and make it easier to digest so it spikes the blood sugar quicker than the whole fruit.
Not natural human food!

Now, as to the quantity of each of the food.
The plate and ¾ of fresh vegetables is nothing short of life saving foods.
No diet offers so much healthy foods in the ratio to meat.
The ratios are taken from nature itself.
You will find that there is a minimum of 7 eatable vegetables to one protein source.
Hence the 7 to 1 servings of vegetables to protein.

As for fruit, we have to remember that while fruit is natural human food.

We have changed the way we grow fruit. Due to crop rotation, transportation and massive commerce – you can now get a banana in December in Alaska!

We would have never been able to get all this fruit all year in the natural world. So fruit is great in season and not part of any meal.

Good for snacking.
As are nuts and seeds.

Oddly, when you look at that list of foods,
you will also see that they are food that
help a horde of health issues.
Stabilize blood sugar, reduce
inflammation, increase energy, reduce
bloating, gas and digestion troubles.
Help keep weight in control and lead to
overall better health in general.
Is it sexy?
No

Is it easy to find outside your home?
No

Is it mass marketed to you?
No
and that is the point.
When you are eating this way.
You are eating to live.
Food is not entertainment.
It is not a distraction or a reward or an
event or attached to anything other than
feeling healthy!

After a week eating this way, cravings
reduce.
You feel lighter.
You may lose some weight but what you
will lose is inflammation.

Bloating.
The highs and lows of the blood sugar
roller coaster.
Feeling tired after meals.
And you will start to understand how food
makes you feel.

How you have been suffering after meals
for years.
Your bowel movements will become more
regular.
Your sleep will not be as disrupted.
And when you slip and eat some non
human foods?
You will notice an unwelcome difference.
And that should help you stay the course
with the plan.

Overall you will be eating more and
consuming less.

You will not miss a meal.
You will be full but feel comfortable.

It will be a very different eating
experience from before. And that
difference might be hard to get use to.

You might find this notion hard to believe
but in the beginning of this adventure, you
will miss feeling bad.

The physical ques of bloating and distended gut that you now see as the reason to stop eating will be absent and you will miss them.
This absence will be misinterpreted as hunger.

The good news is that – that feeling will pass too. Often people start to feel more energized after meals.

The time you use to spend waiting to feel better is now free time to use living!
Doing!
Enjoying the rest of your day.

And in due time, after about 6 months of this way of living. The last thing you will want to do is go back to the treadmill of craving, indulgence and suffering.

**You will know that you are doing good for yourself and our world. That your priorities have become the right ones. That you have done something that few people ever do in their whole lives -
you have put food in its place! And kicked it out of all those part of your life that it never belonged to begin with.**

TWELVE

A world out of balance

We live in a world that is completely out of
balance.
Food and the industries that drive it have
taken over too much of our lives.
Moved into areas of our existence that it
dose not belong. Supplanted the places
where we should be getting joy from.
Replaced feeling of happiness from
interactions and general living with
chemical impostors versions of emotions.
Forced us to accept that food should be in
our minds for every waking hour, all our
lives.

No one has ever told you to put food in its
place.

We have become like Bubba from the
movie Forest Gump – talking endlessly
about all the way to cook shrimp!

We have let this become too much of our
lives.
We are out of balance.

Now, when thinking about the food I have told you is human food, you might start to think, after a time, that it is also a drastic change. That eating only these foods is out of balance.

This will be a sign that you are being pulled back into the matrix of food life. You will have well meaning friends and family that tell you - you can not eat this way forever.
That you deserve a treat. Or that it is just one meal or snack or whatever.

The very hardest part about this is that changing ones life sometimes comes at the cost of other things.
You can not let these arguments set you back. And always remember that every soda you do not drink is a plastic bottle that is not floating in the ocean or poisoning your body.
That fast food restaurants are serving hot plates of death and training children to kill themselves with non food.

That the way you live now is with nature and therefore in balance. And that the world around is the thing that is out of balance with nature.

They say that the longest journey
beginning with a single step.
And this can be the that first step.

And even if you feel lone in those steps,
taking them is the most important thing
you will ever do for your health.

I have spent the last 26 years talking
about this very thing. I have consultant
with 40,000 people on their health.
I have read and learned everything I can
on the subjects of natural health and clean
food and historic and indigenous diets.
I have met and interviewed authors and
doctors and health advocates from all
walks of life.
All manner of health care modalities.
And I was raised by a grandmother that
was a herbalist and one of the original so
called "health nuts".

My experience in this area is a unique one.
One that has lead me to seek out truth,
regardless of dogma or conventional
wisdom. I have taken in all the diets and
ideas and concepts from both sides of
health care.
And I found all of them had one very basic
flaw.
They had more concepts and ideas than
facts!

And even with all this good advice, input
and wisdom from all of my life's journey –
I still became a food addict.
And I still struggle with making the right
choices – everyday.
However, As my father use to say

"knowing is half the battle".

So now you know.
You will be tempted to dismiss this content
as "just one mans opinion" but asked
yourself this one question.
What herein is a lie?
There are none.
The facts and numbers are all real.
The effects of mistakes in food and
commerce are all true.
The industries need for your ignorance
may be distasteful to you but it is very
real.
And lastly, you may not like the tone or
the way I have explained it. The words I
have used.
Or you may even think I have some
agenda as yet undisclosed.

It doesn't matter. Truth is truth.

So, again, now you know.

So, what will you do?

I will leaving you with a summation of my whole life's work.
Three simple lines that can guide you if you get lost in the mess that is our reality.

And with all my heart, I hope it helps you.

These I referee to as:

HENDRY'S 3 LAWS FOR HUMANS

1) Never accept any argument that is made in flavor of a chemical and against nature.

2) Never accept trading off moments of bliss for years of pain.

3) Protect your body and your world – you only get one.

Be Well
RHH